THE PORTABLE BACK SCHOOL
a home study program for proper back care

RAY C. MULRY, Ph.D.
Clinical Psychology
Eisenhower Medical Center,
Rancho Mirage, California

ARTHUR H. WHITE, M.D.
Orthopaedic Surgery,
San Francisco, California

EUGENIA A. KLEIN
Editorial Coordinator,
St. Louis, Missouri

Illustrated

The C. V. Mosby Company
ST. LOUIS • TORONTO • LONDON   1981

Copyright © 1981 by The C. V. Mosby Company

All rights reserved. No part of this book may be reproduced in any manner without written permission of the publisher.

Printed in the United States of America

The C. V. Mosby Company
11830 Westline Industrial Drive, St. Louis, Missouri 63141

Library of Congress Cataloging in Publication Data

Mulry, Ray.
   The portable back school.

   1. Backache. 2. Exercise therapy. 3. Relaxation—Therapeutic use. 4. Patient education. I. White, Arthur H., 1938-   . II. Klein, Eugenia A. III. Title. [DNLM: 1. Backache—Therapy. 2. Physical therapy. WE 755 M96lp]
RD768.M84   617'.560622   81-3960
ISBN 0-8016-3597-7   AACR2

TH/CB/CB 9 8 7 6 5 4 3 2 1

PREFACE

What is *The Portable Back School?* *The Portable Back School* consists of ideas, techniques, and procedures directed toward helping you care for your back. *The Portable Back School* is a condensed version of *The Back School*, a comprehensive team approach to the prevention, treatment, and rehabilitation of low back problems. Through your implementation of this "total person" approach to low back problems, you can initiate a home study program for proper back care.

The concepts, information, and techniques of *The Portable Back School* follow accepted medical guidelines and can be implemented within any low back pain prevention, treatment, or rehabilitation program. For maximum results you will use *The Portable Back School* in conjunction with training personnel familiar with The Back School CORE Training Program.

How is *The Portable Back School* used? The components of *The Portable Back School* include:

1. This manual, which provides you with medical, psychological, exercise, body mechanics, and body movement principles. As you learn to apply this information, you will develop the knowledge and skills essential to the intelligent care of your back.
2. The Personal Concerns Inventory: a self-study, stress-monitoring instrument that will help you identify stressors causing you daily tensions. The specifics for how to use the Personal Concerns Inventory are contained in Chapter 3.
3. Two Relaxation Therapy cassette tapes: each side of each tape contains a 30-minute Relaxation Therapy procedure.

If you do not own a tape player and headphones, you will need to purchase them. Also, you will want to purchase a jack for your headphones so they will fit into your tape player.

Chapter 4 contains specific information on how to do Relaxation Therapy.

Be sure to read this manual thoroughly and initiate your personal program as detailed in the ensuing chapters. Do not rush yourself; be prepared to learn an orderly sequence of ideas regarding how you can help yourself.

Ray C. Mulry
Arthur H. White

CONTENTS

1 Know your back, 7
2 Identify your program, 20
3 Measure your personal concerns, 23
4 Manage your tension, 32
5 Strengthen and stretch your body, 36

1 KNOW YOUR BACK

In order to maintain a healthy back you should understand the importance of balance, muscle strength, body mechanics, tension management, muscle stretching, and rest.

BALANCE

Balance is a most important fundamental principle of body movement. The following illustrations show how balance is used in activities of daily living: pushing and/or pulling (Fig. 1), reaching (Fig. 2), bending or lifting (Fig. 3), twisting (Fig. 4), sitting (Fig. 5), lying (Fig. 6), and standing and/or walking (Fig. 7).

Your spine should be maintained in good balance as much of the time as possible. If you are swayback, hunchback, or overweight or spend long periods of time in awkward working positions, your spine is not in balance. This causes excessive wear on some portion of your spine. The rule for good balance of the spine is to pull in your stomach, tuck your buttocks under, and bend your knees. This is called the *Pelvic Tilt* (Fig. 8). Your shoulders should not be allowed to sag too far forward, nor should they be thrown backward in a military position because this causes a swayback. The abdominal muscles should be tightened and pulled in, thus flattening the swayback. The head should be in a straight line with the spine, not in a forwardly protruding position.

If your spine has been out of balance for long periods, you should consciously realign your body many times throughout the working day. If you sit at a desk all day or work in a bent over position, change your position frequently. Stand up straight to balance the spine, stretch, and move around.

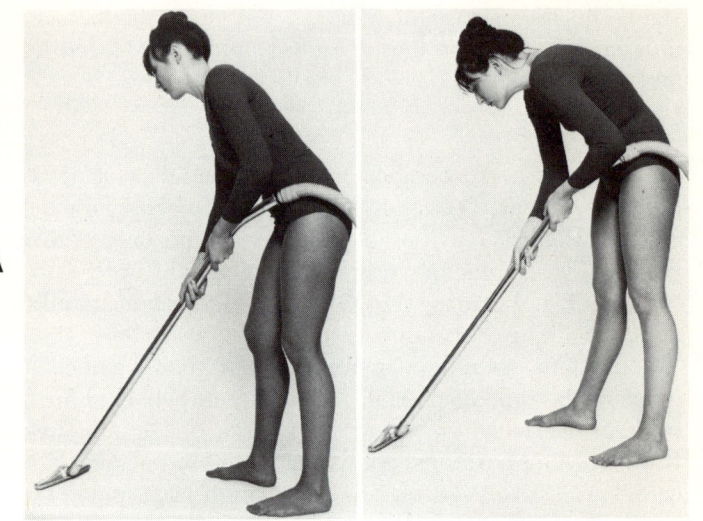

Fig. 1. Pushing and/or pulling.
   A, Right: back straight, stomach in, buttocks under, and knees bent.
   B, Wrong: back bent and knees locked.

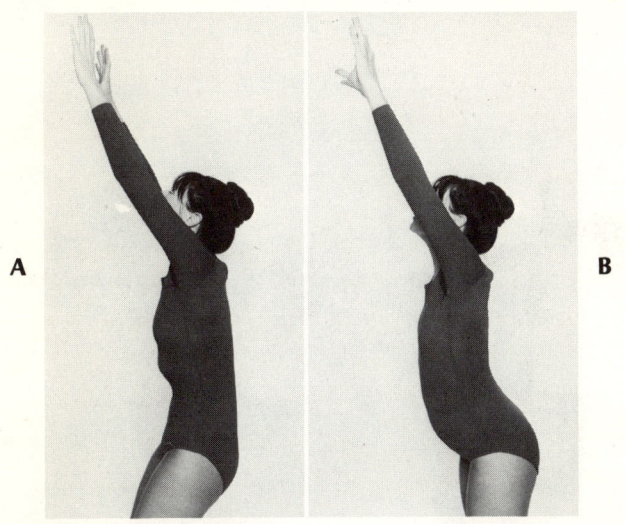

Fig. 2. Reaching.
   A, Right: back straight, stomach in, and buttocks under.
   B, Wrong: swayback.

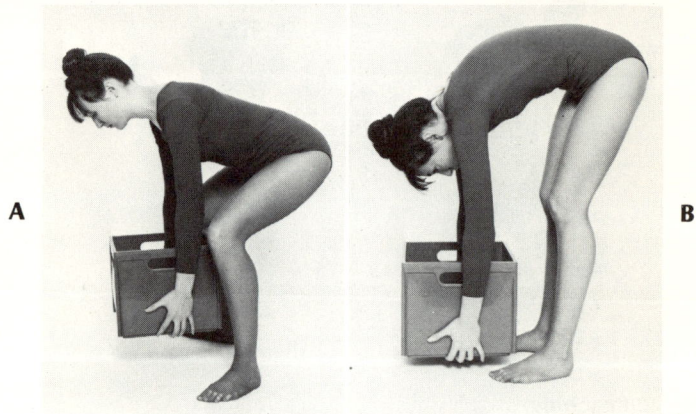

Fig. 3. Bending or lifting.
   A, Right: back straight, stomach in, buttocks under, and knees bent.
   B, Wrong: back bent and knees straight.

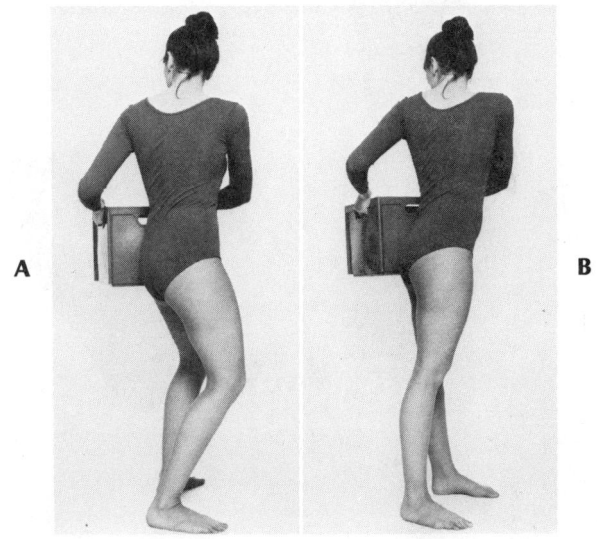

Fig. 4. Twisting.
   A, Right: turn shoulders, hips, and foot together.
   B, Wrong: feet planted and shoulders not in line with hips and feet.

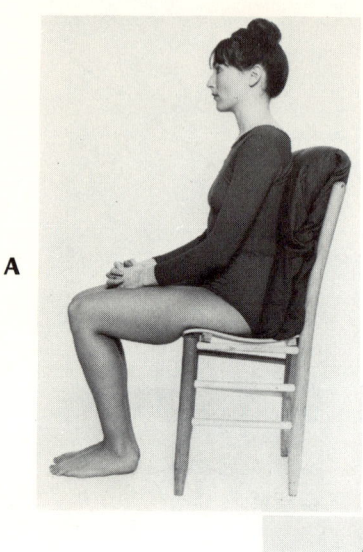
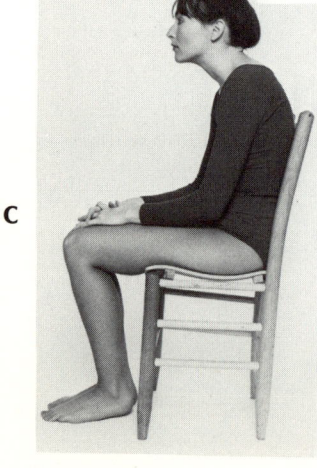

Fig. 5. Sitting.
  A and B, Right: low back supported and straight.
  C, Wrong: back bent.

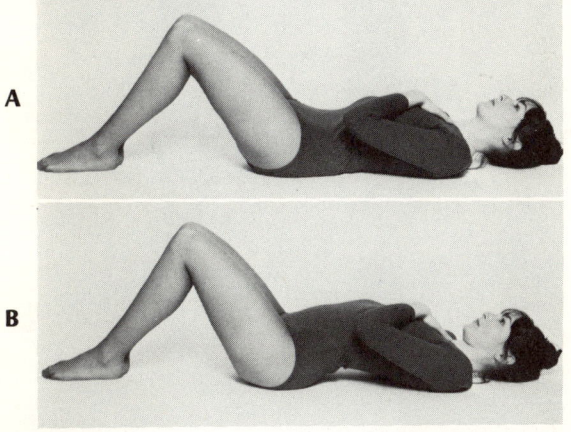

Fig. 6. Lying.
  A, Right: back straight and knees bent.
  B, Wrong: back swayed.

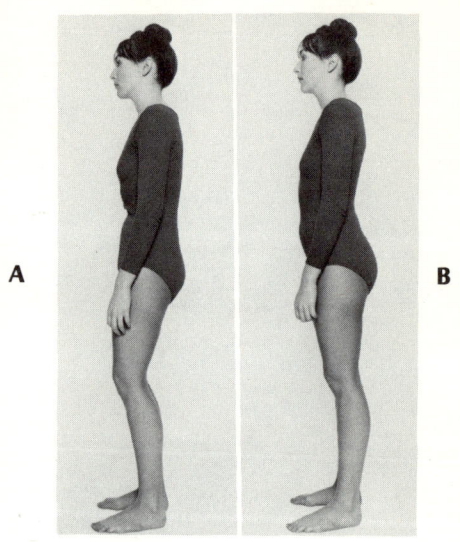

Fig. 7. Standing and/or walking.
  A, Right: back straight, stomach in, buttocks under, and knees bent.
  B, Wrong: swayback and knees straight.

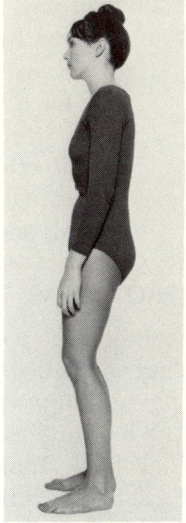

Fig. 8. Pelvic Tilt: back straight, stomach in, buttocks tucked under, and knees bent.

MUSCLE STRENGTHENING

In addition to habits of protective body mechanics and balanced body movements, you want to increase the strength of muscle groups responsible for proper support of the spine. All joints are protected by surrounding muscles, and your spinal column is no exception.

The lower back is protected by four major muscle groups. When these muscles are properly developed, your lower back will have greater protection in activities of daily living. These muscle groups include:

1. *Gluteal* or *buttock* muscles. These are strengthened when you tighten your buttocks as outlined in Exercises 1 and 2 (Chapter 5).
2. *Quadriceps* or *thigh* muscles. These are strengthened through the Wall Slide Hold as outlined in Exercise 3 (Chapter 5).
3. *Abdominal* or *stomach* muscles. These are strengthened through the Partial Sit-up as outlined in Exercise 4 (Chapter 5).

4. *Paraspinal* muscles, or muscles that parallel the spinal column. Because paraspinal muscles are typically well developed and frequently tight, a strengthening exercise for this muscle group is not recommended. However, Stretching Exercises 9, 10, and 11 in Chapter 5 will effectively lead to longer and more flexible paraspinal muscles and thus create greater flexibility of body movement in general.

PROTECTIVE BODY MECHANICS

Protective body mechanics is the use of the most efficient and advantageous body positions as safeguards against physical injury in the performance of physical tasks. There are four protective body mechanics:
1. Back straight
2. Stomach tightened
3. Buttocks tucked under
4. Knees bent

Keeping the back straight normally implies maintaining the spine in an upright or vertical position.

When the stomach muscles are tightened during a task, they support the spine from the front of the body. When you use stomach (abdominal) muscles to support the spine from the front, you are compressing the stomach against the spine to prevent bending of the spine.

Buttocks tucked under means just that. When you tighten your buttocks, you bring your lower spine into a straight line position.

Keeping the knees bent allows the legs to serve as shock absorbers for the spine when you are lifting, moving, or accepting loads (weight) and can lessen the physical strain on the spine.

These basic protective maneuvers in body mechanics are called the Pelvic Tilt. The Pelvic Tilt is recognized in a posture that demonstrates all four protective body mechanics. In general the Pelvic Tilt serves to correct poor posture and is employed as basic protection for the spine in various body movements (Fig. 9).

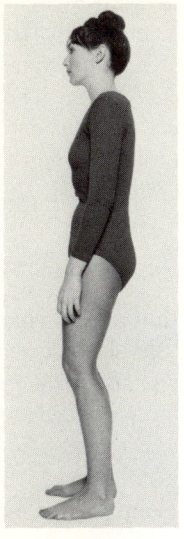
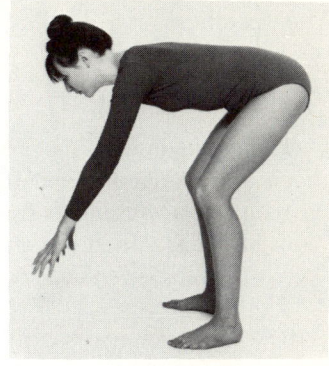

Fig. 9   **Fig. 10**

Fig. 9. Pelvic Tilt: back straight, stomach in, buttocks tucked under, and knees bent.

Fig. 10. Straight Backbend: stomach tightened, back straight, and knees bent.

Although protective body mechanics normally implies maintaining the spine in an upright or vertical position, this is not always possible. There are situations, such as when removing packages from the trunk of a car, that require another kind of protective maneuver. This is called the *Straight Backbend*. (Fig. 10).

The Pelvic Tilt and the Straight Backbend are two basic protective maneuvers, both based on fundamental body mechanics. Between these two protective maneuvers, you should be able to perform most physical tasks without unusual wear or strain on your low back.

TENSION MANAGEMENT

Stress and tension play large parts in all of our lives. When you are stressed, angry, or generally frustrated, muscles can become tight or tense. Tension management is a program that teaches you how to identify stress in your life, how to achieve low levels of physical tension, and how to relax your muscles. Chapters 3 and 4 provide the specifics for a detailed and personalized program of tension management.

MUSCLE STRETCHING

The spine has a range of motion that allows you to move freely. To maintain this mobility you should follow a regular program of stretching exercises. Never use stretching positions for daily activities such as reaching, bending, or lifting.

REST

Rest does not necessarily mean sleep. There are times when you want to rest your muscles; then your spine will need another kind of support. You can rest your spine any time of the day. When sitting use a reclining or contour chair or a straight chair with pillows supporting your back (Fig. 11). When standing you can rest your spine by leaning against the wall in the Pelvic Tilt (Fig. 12). When you lie down, you should be on your side in the contour position or on your back with a pillow under your knees. If you lie on your side, place a pillow under your waist to keep the spine from sagging (Fig. 13).

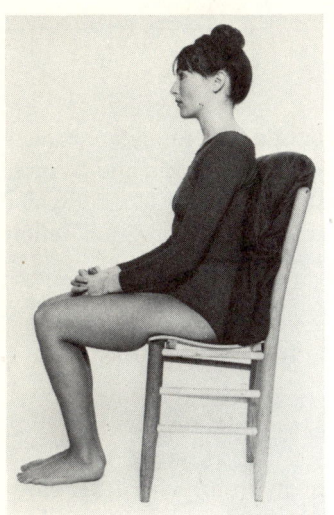 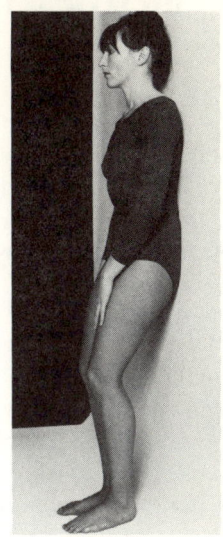

Fig. 11   **Fig. 12**

Fig. 11. Sitting rest position. Right way to sit with low back supported and straight.
Fig. 12. Standing rest position.

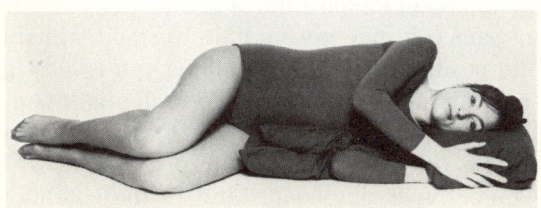

Fig. 13. Lying rest position.

2 IDENTIFY YOUR PROGRAM

To help you identify your program, the following categories have been established: new pain, old pain, and no pain. Check the symptoms in these categories to see which apply to you. After you have identified your program, follow the prescribed treatment plan.

NEW PAIN PROGRAM

Symptoms:
Any new low back pain
Shooting leg pain, numbness, tingling, weakness

Treatment:
Your pain will probably go away in a few weeks. However, once you have had back pain, you will most likely have a recurrence. Therefore the following treatment plan is of critical importance:

1. Lie down in your most comfortable position. This is a contour position on your side or back (Fig. 13). Stay in this position as much of the time as possible. It sometimes takes several hours in the proper position for the pain to subside.

2. Change positions slowly. Tighten your stomach muscles before moving. Roll on your side and push yourself to an upright position as painlessly as possible. Sit as little as possible. Stand in the position of greatest comfort. Because of your pain you may not be able to stand straight. Give in to the position your body is telling you is least painful. Walk only for short distances to go to the bathroom or get something to eat. Return to the lying position that is most comfortable. Stay as free of pain as possible.

3. Contact your physician. Most of the conditions that cause new back pain are potentially serious and will need the direction and aid of a physician. There are many things

that a physician can do to help resolve this pain more safely and rapidly.

4. Start immediately to practice Relaxation Therapy at least once a day. This will help reduce tension, which contributes to back pain (see Chapter 4).

5. After you are able to function without pain medication, you can return to the normal activities of daily living (see Chapter 1). You should sit, stand, and walk only in the correct positions. Increase your activities painlessly without the use of pain medication.

6. Begin your recovery program with Exercises 1, 2, 3, and 4 (see Chapter 5). Do these painlessly. If they cause pain, stop doing them and seek the attention of your physician or Back School instructor. You should be able to move around the house in a pain-controlled condition and take short walks and limited drives in the car.

7. When you can painlessly perform Exercises 1 to 4 as prescribed, add Exercises 5, 6, 7, and 8 to your routine (see Chapter 5). If they cause any pain, stop immediately. The following day there may be some muscle soreness, but there should not be any increase in your back pain or spread of your back pain in any direction. You should now be ready to go back to office work, do housework, participate in some recreational activities such as swimming and bicycling, resume sexual activity, and travel.

8. When you have been pain-free for 3 months, you may advance from this program to the No Pain Program.

OLD PAIN PROGRAM

Symptoms:
   Mainly moderate low back pain
   Recurrence of minor symptoms
Treatment:
Your back pain is not likely to disappear spontaneously. You will have to make some major changes in what you do with and for your body on a daily basis.

1. Learn and use all of the balance and body movements in Chapter 1.

2. Initiate an ongoing program of tension management (see Chapters 3 and 4). This will help regulate tension that contributes to back pain.

3. Do Exercises 1 to 4 until you have achieved twice the normal recommended levels for Exercises 1 and 2 and until you can maintain a Wall Slide Hold (Exercise 3) for 1 minute and a Partial Sit-up (Exercise 4) for 1 minute.

4. Proceed to Exercises 5 to 8 (see Chapter 5). Your pain should decrease by following the preceding recommendations. If the pain does not decrease, seek the attention of your physician.

5. When you have been pain-free in normal daily activities for several months, you may add Exercises 9 to 11, as long as you are able to do them painlessly. There is a limit to what your back will allow you to do. You should be able to swim, bicycle, play tennis, and play golf. Renewed pain will tell you when you may be doing these activities improperly. Speak with your physician or Back School instructor.

NO PAIN PROGRAM

Symptoms:
  None
  Possible vague low back discomfort or concern for physical fitness and prevention of back pain

Treatment:

1. You are pain-free and want to stay fit. Review body mechanics and the balanced body movements in Chapter 1. You can probably do Exercises 1 to 11 completely (see Chapter 5). Do them slowly. Do not overexert. Immediately stop doing any exercises that cause pain.

2. Maximum success in this exercise routine will require an ongoing program of tension management (see Chapters 3 and 4). Starting today practice Relaxation Therapy once a day and complete your Personal Concerns Inventory on a daily basis.

3 MEASURE YOUR PERSONAL CONCERNS

STRESS AND TENSION IN EVERYDAY LIFE

When you are having trouble with your back, it is important to remember you are not just muscles, bones, and nerves. You are also a feeling human being, and emotions are as important to the care of your back as anything else. When you are happy, joyful, relaxed, and full of buoyant feelings, you move with greater flexibility and ease. On the other hand, when you feel angry, depressed, tense, and burdened with frustrations and personal concerns, you tighten up, restrict yourself, and struggle with the world around you. When you examine your life-style through the use of the Personal Concerns Inventory (PCI), you will readily identify a variety of potential stressors that can make you tense; noise pollution, financial pressures, problems with children, marital problems, time pressures, medical bills, and trouble with your employer are a few potential stressors.

Stress is a most important concept and one that has considerable bearing on your health. For example, anything that makes your heart work beyond normal, makes you perspire, or causes your muscles to tighten may be considered a stressor.

There are two kinds of stress. *Positive stress* is any influence that disrupts bodily balance and leads to a strengthening of physical functioning. If you go jogging, your heart rate will typically increase, you will perspire, and your muscles will tighten. If you exercise intelligently, you will make your body stronger and healthier.

Negative stress is any influence that disrupts bodily balance and leads to a weakening of physical functioning. For example, if you jog beyond your limits, you may damage

PERSONAL CONCERNS
A Program

DATE _____

SEX _____ AGE _____ HEIGHT _____ WEIGHT _____

MARITAL STATUS _____

	DAY 1	DAY 2	DAY 3	DAY 4	DAY 5	DAY 6	DAY 7	TOTAL	DAY 1	DAY 2
Need More Recreation										
Noise At Home										
Noise At Work										
Sleeping Problems										
Chest Pain										
Problems With Children										
Weight Problem										
Need to be More Assertive										
Recent Death in Family										
High Blood Pressure										
Conflicts With Relatives										
Poor Eating Habits										
Short Temper										
Freeway Traffic										
Cigarette Smoking										
Feel Guilty										
Back Pain										
Alcohol (self)										
Alcohol (other)										
Jealousy										
Pill Consumption										
Boredom										
Tension										
Worry Too Much										
Medical Bills										
Need Employment										
Divorce										
Separation										
Dislike Job										
Continued Physical Pain										
Job Security										
Unexpressed Anger										
Headaches										
Trouble Making Decisions										
Conflicts With Neighbors										
Marital Problems										
Financial Difficulties										
Desire More Social Life										
Need to Relax										
Trouble With Employer										
Need Physical Exercise										
Need Friends										
Nervousness										
Sex Difficulties										
More Time for Myself										
Deadlines on Job										
Depression										
Can't Say No										
Ulcers										
Loneliness										
General Unhappiness										
More Self-discipline										
TOTAL										

Fig. 14

INVENTORY
of Self-Study

USING THE FOLLOWING SCALE, CONSIDER EACH ISSUE AND INDICATE TO WHAT DEGREE THAT ISSUE IS A CONCERN TO YOU ON A DAY TO DAY BASIS.

SCALE
0 — 1 — 2 — 3 — 4 — 5 — 6 — 7 — 8 — 9 — 10
LITTLE   MODERATELY   VERY MUCH

DAY 3	DAY 4	DAY 5	DAY 6	DAY 7	TOTAL	DAY 1	DAY 2	DAY 3	DAY 4	DAY 5	DAY 6	DAY 7	TOTAL

or weaken your body and, of course, your general condition of health. What you want in your daily life is a desirable amount of positive stress and no negative stress.

DEVELOPING STRESSOR IDENTIFICATION SKILLS

Stress and tension play important roles in the care of your back, and it is important to learn how to identify those aspects in your life that are stressful for you. This is called *developing stressor identification skills.* To help you identify stressors the PCI lists 52 items that are potential trouble spots (Fig. 14). Through the daily use of this inventory you will learn which stressors are causing you concern on a given day and which concerns persist from one day to the next. Those concerns are the important ones, especially if they are consistently given high ratings (i.e., 7, 8, 9, or 10).

Your daily ratings for each item should be made at the end of the day and should reflect your experience on that day. You may be unsure which rating to start with on a specific item. That does not matter because *you are free to change your mind the next day and to increase or decrease your rating as you feel it accurately represents your true concern.*

As each item is presented, read the brief description of what that item refers to and insert your rating in the space provided. If you are unsure whether or not you are concerned with a specific item, just ask yourself *if the issue causes you tension and or worry.* If it does not, you may assign it a rating of zero.

1. Need More Recreation _____
Are you concerned about your need for recreational (fun/play) time?

2. Noise At Home _____
Does the noise level at home bother you? Have you noticed this before as a potential source of tension? Does the noise from traffic, airplanes, television, voices, dogs barking, or other such sounds bother you?

3. Noise At Work _____
Is your work situation quiet and pleasant, or is noise, (typewriters, voices, traffic, hammering) a factor in your daily personal balance?

4. Sleeping Problems _____
Did you sleep well last night? Did you use sleeping aids? Were you rested when you woke up?

5. Chest Pain _____
Have you noticed any pain in your chest today? If so, are you concerned about it?

6. Problems With Children _____
Of course, you care about your children, but have you been *concerned* or *worried* about them *today*?

7. Weight Problem _____
Are you the right weight for your good health? Did your weight bother or concern you today?

8. Need To Be More Assertive _____
Did you let opportunity slip by because you were too passive to stand up for yourself? If so, does this concern you?

9. Recent Death In Family _____
It is possible you have recently experienced a death in the family, and it is also possible this does not concern you. Be honest with yourself and rate the item appropriately.

10. High Blood Pressure _____
Do you know your blood pressure? If so, does it concern you?

11. Conflicts With Relatives _____
Have relatives (other than your spouse or children) been a source of tension for you today?

12. Poor Eating Habits _____
Do you eat regularly and maintain a healthy diet?

13. Short Temper _____
Did you find yourself particularly on edge today? Did you lose your temper?

14. Freeway Traffic _____
Did the noise, congestion, speed, and general activity on

the highway bother you today? (This item is particularly relevant for urban communities.)

15. Cigarette Smoking _____
Are you a smoker? Does this concern you? This does not refer to someone else's smoking because there is very little you can do about that.

16. Feel Guilty _____
Did you experience guilt feelings today? Does this concern you?

17. Back Pain _____
Did you experience back pain today? If so, how important is this to you, and did you do anything about it?

18. Alcohol (self) _____
This refers to your own drinking habits and how well you manage yourself when you are drinking. Even if you did not have a drink today, you may still be concerned about this issue in your personal habits and general tendencies.

19. Alcohol (other) _____
Did someone else's drinking bother you today?

20. Jealousy _____
Did you feel jealous today? If so, does this concern you?

21. Pill Consumption _____
Are you taking pills more than necessary or in a way contrary to medical advice? This does not refer to vitamin pills or any other pill that is prescribed by a physician for a specific medical condition such as diabetes or thyroid problems.

22. Boredom _____
Were you bored today? Was your day rather pointless?

23. Tension _____
Was this a tense day for you? Did your tensions get out of hand?

24. Worry Too Much _____
Did you feel worried today? Is this becoming a concern of yours?

25. Medical Bills _____
Are you concerned about accumulating medical bills?

26. Need Employment _____
Are you concerned about finding a job?

27. Divorce _____
Did you have thoughts about an ongoing or pending divorce today? Is this a concern of yours?

28. Separation _____
Did you have thoughts about an ongoing or pending separation today? Is this a concern of yours?

29. Dislike Job _____
Did your work situation annoy you today? Do you feel satisfied with what you are doing in your job?

30. Continued Physical Pain _____
Has a continuing pain such as headache, backache, or chest pain been on your mind today?

31. Job Security _____
Do you feel secure in your job?

32. Unexpressed Anger _____
Are you concerned about angry feelings that you keep inside?

33. Headaches _____
Did you have a headache today? Are you concerned about this?

34. Trouble Making Decisions _____
Do you go back and forth and find it difficult to take decisive action?

35. Conflicts With Neighbors _____
Are the neighbors getting on your nerves?

36. Marital Problems _____
Are you and your spouse getting along? If not, how much does this concern you? If you are not married, you may relate this item to an important ongoing interpersonal relationship.

37. Financial Difficulties _____
Did money pressures bother you today?

38. Desire More Social Life _____
Do you feel the need for more leisure time with others?

39. Need To Relax _____
Are you attending to your need for relaxation? Is this something you postpone?

40. Trouble With Employer _____
Are your working relationships satisfactory?

41. Need Physical Exercise _____
Are you aware of your needs for adequate physical exercise?

42. Need Friends _____
Are you concerned about feelings of friendship? Did this issue surface for you today?

43. Nervousness _____
Were your nerves on edge today?

44. Sex Difficulties _____
Are you concerned about the adequacy of your sex life?

45. More Time For Myself _____
Do you feel the need to be alone and pursue your own interests?

46. Deadlines On Job _____
Did deadlines and time pressures get to you at work?

47. Depression _____
Did you feel down and depressed today?

48. Can't Say No _____
Did you find yourself doing things you did not want to do because you were unable to say no to someone?

49. Ulcers _____
Were you concerned about ulcers today?

50. Loneliness _____
Did you feel lonely and in need of people in your life today?

51. General Unhappiness _____
When you take all things into consideration, do you feel your life is generally in balance?

52. More Self-discipline _____
Very little changes for the better unless you exert yourself in a growth-oriented manner. Are you doing what you need to do to bring your life into balance?

Now that you have made 52 self-assessments, add them up to determine your *total personal concerns score*. Each day, as you total your PCI ratings, you can see whether your overall level is increasing, decreasing, or staying the same. The goal, of course, is to lower your score as much as possible.

The next step in your self-analysis is to identify *primary* and *secondary* personal concerns. First, go through all 52 PCI ratings and identify all items rated 7, 8, 9, or 10. These are your primary concerns. Secondary concerns have PCI ratings of 3, 4, 5, and 6. These are important issues but are secondary to primary concerns. Ratings of 1 and 2 are viewed as concerns but are not significant enough to require your attention. A rating of zero, of course, indicates no concern and no need for attention to that matter on that day. The primary concerns are your most significant trouble spots and indicate where you can make the most constructive changes in your daily routine. Always take your PCI to Back School and discuss your primary concerns with your instructor.

Now that you have identified and rated your primary concerns, it is important to learn how to reduce your PCI scores through Relaxation Therapy.

4 MANAGE YOUR TENSION

Relaxation Therapy (RT) is a simple technique designed to help reduce tension. It takes about 30 minutes per session. You will need a cassette tape player and headphones. Most headphones may not fit into a cassette tape recorder; therefore you will need to purchase an inexpensive adapter. First, select a quiet, preferably dark room where you are not likely to be interrupted by noise or by the activities of others for at least 30 minutes. Lie *on your back* and close your eyes. Place a couple of *pillows under your knees*, which will help flatten your back. *Do not use a big pillow* under your neck or head. A small pillow under your head or a rolled towel under your neck will give you the support you need (Fig. 15). This will help you relax with your spine in a straight line position. During RT it is possible you will get chilled, so consider using a blanket or some other item to cover your chest. If you are concerned about incoming calls, take the phone off the hook.

RT consists of three basic stages. The *first stage* consists of some basic breathing exercises that help you settle in, but they also prepare you for the overall relaxation experience provided by the RT cassette tapes. It is important that you do not strain yourself during these breathing exercises. Proceed at a pace you are comfortable with and do not concern yourself with whether you are in perfect step with the speaker. You will find your own natural pace, and this is as it should be.

The *second stage* consists of muscle relaxation exercises. Just listen to the tape and don't worry if your mind drifts to other subjects. Just continue to listen to the tape without effort, and you will relax. Stages one and two take about 15 minutes.

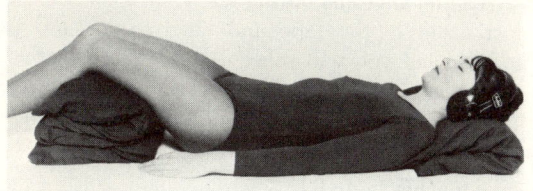

Fig. 15. Position for Relaxation Therapy.

The *third stage* takes 15 minutes. During this stage you will continue your deep relaxation while listening to the sounds of nature.

Incidentally, many people *fall asleep* during RT. This is a good result. Sleep is a form of deep relaxation and something most people with back pain need.

How often can or should I do RT?
You can do RT as often as you like. It cannot harm you.

Should I do RT before I go to sleep at night?
You have undoubtedly heard the advertisements, "Relax and go to sleep." If you want to rid yourself of sleeping pills, RT will be of considerable benefit to you.

Can I relax too deeply and not wake up on my own?
No, your body has its own regulatory system. You will not relax too much, and you will wake up when you are ready.

Is RT the same as biofeedback?
No, but biofeedback is also a process through which you can learn to relax. You may also use biofeedback as another form of therapy. One of the advantages of RT is that the tapes can be used at any time and in the privacy of your home.

Can I also meditate if I want to?
Yes, anything that helps you to relax and feel good about yourself is useful to you.

How long does it take to respond to RT?
Most people respond during their first session. Almost everyone will relax fully in two or three sessions.

Should I try to do anything during RT?
No, just listen to the tape and have a pleasant time. Let yourself go, and you will relax regardless of whether or not you are concentrating on the words and procedures of RT. RT is, in many respects, a *process of letting go*. Do not interfere with this process if you can help it.

Do I need a teacher to do RT?
No, this text is sufficient for your need in this regard. Allow your own experience to be your guide, and learn to trust yourself.

I have been afraid of hypnosis because I don't like not being in "control" of myself. Does this relate to RT in any way?
No! RT emphasizes you and your control over yourself. If you allow yourself to let go and relax, you will.

I often feel guilty when I take time out to relax. What can I do about this?
Remember, you are a more rewarding person to others when you are relaxed, balanced, and free of discomfort. You have a *right to a restful time alone*.

Does RT require any self-discipline?
Yes, it may seem strange to you, but you will have to take time out from your daily schedule to do RT. Self-regulation does require self-discipline.

How long does an RT session last?
Each RT cassette tape lasts 30 minutes. You may continue in a deep state of rest after the tape player shuts off. This will be determined by how much your body is in need of additional rest and relaxation.

Will I always need to use the tape player and the tapes to relax?
No, you will eventually learn how to relax on your own without the tapes. This is one of the *primary reasons* for doing RT on a regular basis. Once you learn "how" to relax, you will be able to apply this skill in everyday situations.

Does it make any difference if I do RT daily?
Yes, RT is a process that helps you help yourself. Daily relaxation is essential to your overall care of yourself. If you are more tense than usual or are in the early stages of caring for your back, you may do RT two or even three times a day. Let

your needs for relaxation be your guide, and don't wait until you are overly tense.

What are the advantages of using headphones?
The headphones have three benefits, but these benefits are not essential to RT: (1) they allow you to do RT so no one else will hear the tape, which is particularly important at bedtime when you are sleeping with someone who desires a quiet environment; (2) headphones help screen out extraneous noise that can disrupt the relaxation process; and (3) headphones provide the listener with a more "real life" reception of the nature sounds, which results in more complete relaxation responses.

However, many people do RT without headphones and have satisfying results.

Is RT the most important part of the total tension management program?
No, tension management is the integration of stressor identification skills with relaxation skills so you will cope more effectively with daily stresses and tensions.

Perhaps the most important aspect of tension management is that you do what needs to be done so you establish effective and lasting solutions to your personal concerns.

Should I develop relaxation skills before I start stretching exercises?
Yes, relaxation skills are very relevant to your developing ability to relax into the stretch. Stretching is a muscle lengthening process that is based, in part, on your ability to let your muscles go into ever more advanced stretches.

5 STRENGTHEN AND STRETCH YOUR BODY

In this chapter you will find the exercises that are keyed to your individual program (see Chapter 2). Follow your program carefully and *do not do any exercise that causes pain.*

EXERCISE 1: Pelvic Tilt on Your Back

1. Lie on your back with your knees bent.
2. Flatten the small of your back by tightening the stomach muscles and tilting your pelvis.
3. Tighten your buttocks.
4. Hold this position for 10 seconds. Repeat 10 times.
5. The Pelvic Tilt will be performed as the first step in each exercise.

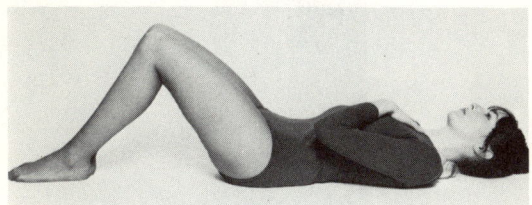

EXERCISE 2: Pelvic Tilt Against the Wall

1. Stand with the small of your back *flat* against the wall.
2. Place your heels 12 inches from the wall.
3. Pull in your stomach.
4. Tighten your buttocks.
5. Bend your knees.
6. Hold this position for 10 seconds. Repeat 10 times.

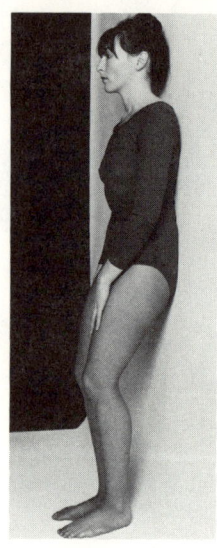

EXERCISE 3: Wall Slide Hold

1. Stand with the small of your back flat against the wall.
2. Place your heels 12 to 18 inches from the wall.
3. Pull in your stomach.
4. Bend your knees and slide 6 to 8 inches down the wall.
5. Hold this position for 10 seconds.
6. Return to the standing position by sliding back up the wall. Repeat 10 times. Relax and walk around between repetitions.
7. Progressively increase your distance down the wall until your thighs are at a 90-degree angle to the wall.
8. The minimum holding time goal at a 90-degree angle is 1 minute.
9. Eventually increase holding time in the 90-degree angle position to 3 minutes.

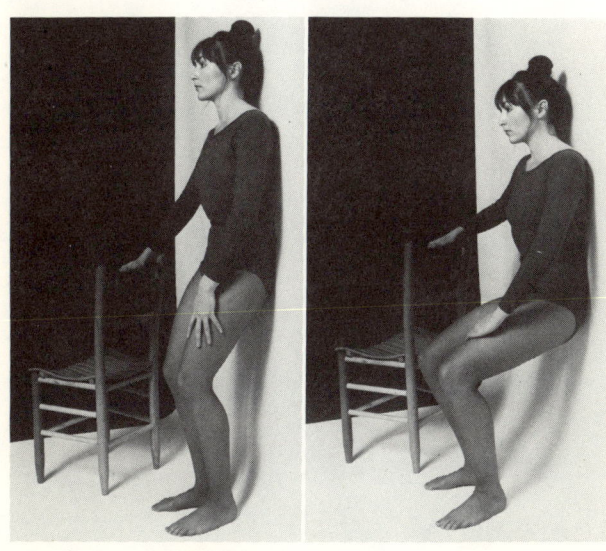

EXERCISE 4: Partial Sit-up

1. Lie on your back with your knees bent and in the Pelvic Tilt.
2. Reach for the top of your knees and lift your shoulder blades off the floor.
3. Hold for a count of 10.
4. Return to the start position and relax.
5. Gradually increase your holding time capacity to 3 minutes.

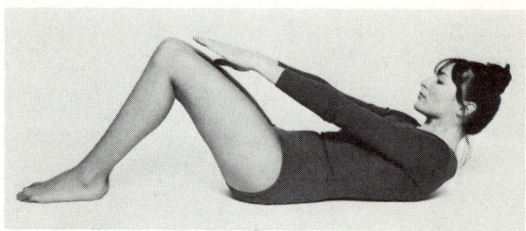

STOP

**DO NOT PROCEED BEYOND THIS POINT
UNLESS YOU ARE ABLE
TO DO EXERCISES 1 TO 4 PAINLESSLY.**

The *stretching* exercises on the following pages have been carefully selected to help you find a systematic method for achieving greater flexibility.

Learning how to stretch properly so you do not injure muscle tissue is essential to this stretching program. Stretch up to the point of pain but not beyond that point.

Relaxation is the first step in stretching. Concentrate on the feeling of relaxation and allow that feeling to spread throughout the muscle group you are about to stretch. *You must learn that straining, bouncing, pulling, and other similar movements have no place in your stretching activities.* Your breathing should be slow and easy and a flowing part of your stretch. In other words, you are engaged in a natural activity that will lead to the relaxed letting go of muscle tissue.

EXERCISE 5: Knee to Chest

1. Lie on your back with your knees bent in the Pelvic Tilt position.
2. Place both hands behind the thigh and pull gently and slowly toward the chest, exhaling as the knee comes up.
3. Relax and hold for a count of five.
4. Release and inhale as the leg returns to the start position.
5. Repeat with the other leg.
6. Do five repetitions with each leg.

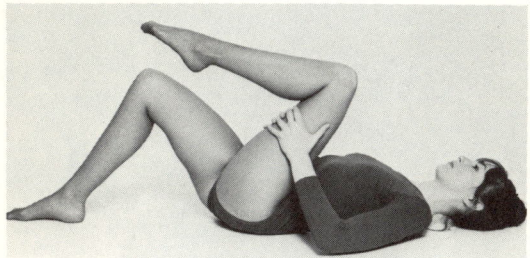

EXERCISE 6: Both Knees to Chest

1. Lie on your back with your knees bent in the Pelvic Tilt position.
2. Place both hands behind your thighs and bring both knees to the chest, exhaling as the knees approach the chest.
3. Relax and hold for a count of five.
4. Release and inhale as your legs return to the start position.
5. Repeat five times.

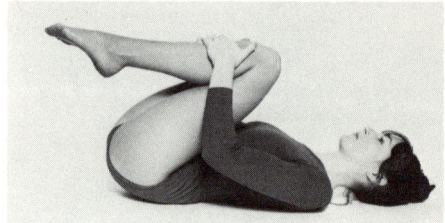

EXERCISE 7: The Hamstring Stretch

1. Lie on your back with your knees bent in the Pelvic Tilt position.
2. Bring one knee *toward your chest,* exhaling as the knee comes up. Reach forward with both hands and hold behind the knee.
3. Straighten your leg upward.
4. Hold for a count of five. Bend the knee and return to the start position.
5. Repeat with the other leg.
6. Do five repetitions with each leg.

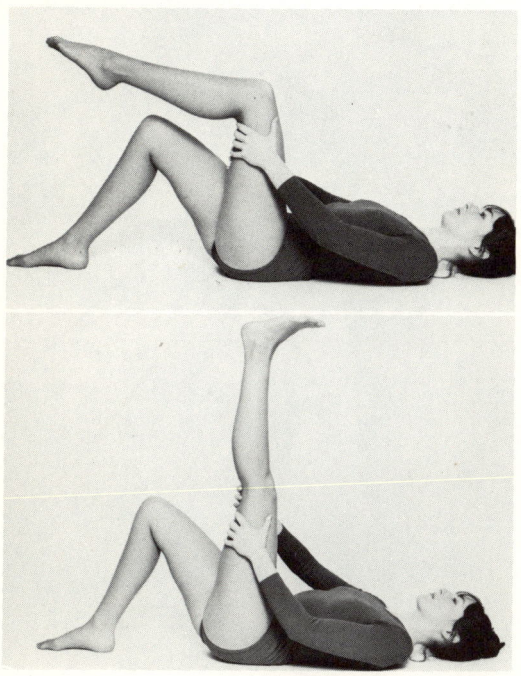

EXERCISE 8: The Heel Cord Stretch

1. At arms length, face the wall, a desk, or other sturdy object.
2. Place one foot 12 inches behind the other with both heels planted firmly on the floor.
3. Lean into the wall or object.
4. Stretch the heel cord and hamstring of the rear leg by leaning forward over the front foot.
5. Hold for 5 seconds.
6. Alternate with the other leg.
7. Do each leg five times.

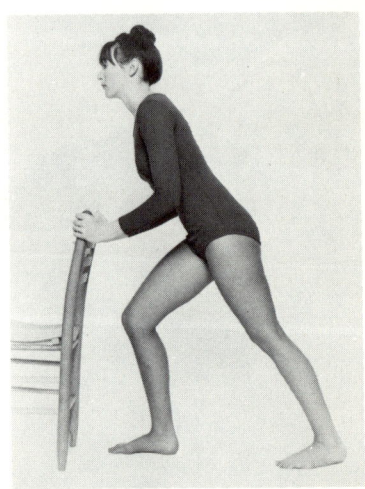

**IF YOU CAN PERFORM ALL
STRENGTHENING AND STRETCHING EXERCISES
CORRECTLY AND PAINLESSLY,
ADD EXERCISES 9 AND 10.**

EXERCISE 9: The Standing Hamstring Stretch

1. Stand up straight with the feet a shoulder's width apart.
2. *Slowly* bend forward at the waist.
3. Let your head, neck, and arms hang freely.
4. Relax into the stretch for 30 seconds.
5. Do not bounce when doing this stretch.
6. *Bend your knees* and return to the standing position.
7. Repeat this exercise and continue the stretch for 45 seconds.
8. Repeat this exercise and continue the stretch for 60 seconds.

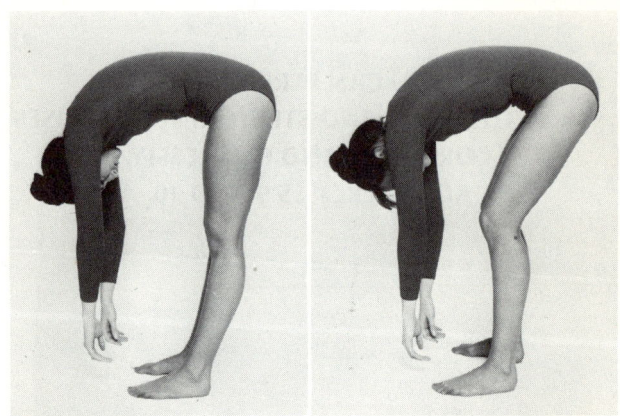

EXERCISE 10: The Full-Body Groin Stretch

1. Sit on the floor and place the soles of the feet together.
2. Grasp your toes and gently pull your heels toward the groin.
3. Place your elbows in front of your shins. Hang your head loosely.
4. Relax into the stretch for 30 seconds
5. Repeat for a 45-second stretch.
6. Repeat for a 60-second stretch.

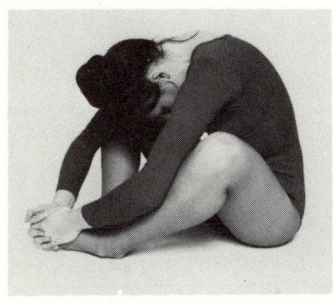

**IF YOU ARE ABLE TO PERFORM
ALL PREVIOUS EXERCISES PAINLESSLY,
ADD EXERCISE 11.**

EXERCISE 11: The Moving Squat

1. Stand with your feet flat, 6 to 9 inches apart, toes pointed out slightly.
2. Squat slowly until your armpits are over your knees.
3. Allow your back to relax, with your head hanging in a relaxed position.
4. Sway slowly from side to side. Next sway slowly forward and backward in a similar manner, then in a circular fashion clockwise and counterclockwise.
5. *Caution:* you may initially have trouble with your balance. Be careful not to fall *backward.*
6. Relax into the stretch for 30 seconds.
7. Repeat for a 45-second stretch.
8. Repeat for a 60-second stretch.

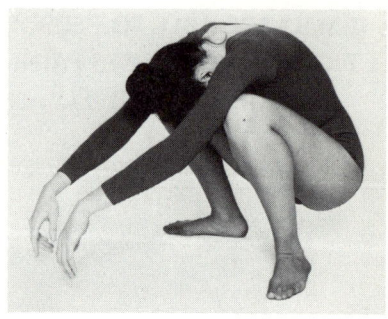

DAILY MAINTENANCE PROGRAM

Proper back care requires a continuing strengthening and stretching exercise program. It is recommended that you follow a Daily Maintenance Program. Do these 11 exercises in the following order, once in the morning and once in the evening:
1. Wall Slide — 3 minutes
2. Partial Sit-up — 3 minutes
3. Moving Squat — 30 seconds
4. The Standing Hamstring Stretch — 30 seconds
5. The Full-Body Groin Stretch — 30 seconds
6. Repeat the Moving Squat — increase to 45 seconds
7. Repeat the Standing Hamstring Stretch — increase to 45 seconds
8. Repeat the Full-Body Groin Stretch — increase to 45 seconds
9. Repeat the Moving Squat — increase to 60 seconds
10. Repeat the Standing Hamstring Stretch — increase to 60 seconds
11. Repeat the Full-Body Groin Stretch — increase to 60 seconds

The Moving Squat and the Standing Hamstring Stretch can be done at any time during the day to counteract muscle tightness.

Remain relaxed. Relaxation leads to stretching, and stretching leads to relaxation. Never push or rush yourself while stretching. The quality of the stretch is far more important than the number of stretches.